SIRTFOOD DIET RECIPE BOOK

The complete Diet Guide with Delicious Recipes to Lose Weight fast, Burn Fat, get Lean and improve your life.

Stephanie Smith

Disclaimer Notice

Please note that every information shared in the course of this book is for educational and entertainment purposes only. Efforts have been made to ensure every information is accurate, reliable, and up to date is given. Readers yield that every information rendered by the author is in the course of providing legal, financial, professional, or medical advice. The information shared in this book has been collected from various sources. Do ensure to contact a professional or expert before engaging in any technique given in this book.

By reading this document, the user agrees that the author is not liable for any loss, whether directly or indirectly, from the use of information shared in this document, including errors, inaccuracies, or omissions.

Content

Pan-Fried Salmon Fillet with Caramelized Endive, Arugula & Celery Leaf Salad

Butternut Squash and Date Tagine with Buckwheat Buckwheat Noodles In A Miso Broth with Kale,Celery & Tofu

Strawberry Buckwheat Tabbouleh

Buckwheat Pasta Salad

Waldorf Salad

Sirt Salad

Aromatic Chicken Breast With Kale and Red Onions and A Tomato and Chili Salsa

Turkey Escalope with Sage, Capers, and Parsley and Spiced Cauliflower

Sirt Omelete

Harissa and Baked Tofu with Cauliflower Mushroom and Tofu Scramble

Tuscan Beans Stew and Buckwheat Noodles

Char-Grilled Beef With Onion Rings, Red Wine Jus, Kale, Garlic, and Herb-Roasted Potatoes

Spiced Scrambled Eggs

Roasted Eggplants Wedges with Walnut and Parsley Pesto and Tomato Salad

Tofu and Shiitake Mushroom Soup

Smoked Salmon Pasta with Chili and Arugula

Sirt Chili Con Carne

Butter Beans and Miso Dip With Oatcakes and Celery Sticks

Kidney Beans Mole with Baked Potatoes

Kale Curry and Chicken with Bombay Potatoes

Baked Chicken Breast with Walnut and Parsley Pesto and Red Onion Salad

Sirt Blueberry Pancake

Mushroom Scrambled Eggs

Sirt Smoked Salmon Omelet
PHASE TWO RECIPES
Strawberry, Celery & Watermelon Juice Green Juice
Instant Coconut Iced Coffee

INTRODUCTION

Sirtfood was introduced first in 2016 and has become a trendy new diet, especially with celebrities. According to its creators, Sirtfood is a unique diet and works by stimulating some protein called sirtuin. When taken, these foods can help cut back on calories without creating an energy shortage to activate the skinny gene.

Sirtuin is said to influence the body's ability to cut out fats while reducing the body's metabolic reaction towards creating body weight. They, therefore, decrease the body fat at the same time maintaining the body muscles. However, many researchers doubt that sirtuin improves the skeletal muscles and glycogen formation.

The Sirtfood Diet contains chemicals that trigger genes similar to those caused by fasting and exercise. This chemical is called polyphenols. It activates sirtuins, which are said to control metabolism, moods, and ageing examples are the likes of red wine, spinach, and chocolate. Food like fresh mango, red onions, turmeric, and cinnamon are also great Sirtfood. A diet rich in sirtuin can cause weight loss and provide the individual with optimum health without compromising muscle.

Include a healthy Sirt Diet in your meals to lower calories, weight gain, and lead to vibrant health and sustainability. Change from your strenuous fat burning routines and prevents diseases from taking charge of your body by following the diet developed by food professionals who have proven the impact of Sirtfood.

Food like dark chocolate, coffee, and kale are food that triggers the body's skinny gene. And, Sirtfood provides an avenue where you can eat healthily for weight loss, with its easy to make, delicious recipes, and long-term maintenance plan. Also, Sirt diet is for everybody, and the meals are easily accessible and affordable. It is one diet that allows you to enjoy tasty delicacies while taking its toll on the fat cells.

According to this Sirtfood program, consuming these foods will activate the skinny gene, which will trim down your body fat up to seven kilograms in a matter of seven days.

WHAT IS THE SIRT FOOD

Sirt food is meals induced with ingredients that contain sirtuin. Sirtuins are a class of proteins that defend our body cells from dying and prevent diseases. They also help regulate the body's metabolic actions, enhance the growth of muscles, and increase fat loss abilities.

Who Developed Sirt Food Diet

Sirtfood diet was established by the famous writer and wellness experts, Aidan Goggins and Glen Matten. Both nutritionists focused on administering good health rather than weight loss through their diet.

Things You Can Eat On The Sirt Food Diet

All Sirtfood diets are focused on giving you healthy food intake. Some of these healthy food are:

Red wine
Dark chocolate Apples
Walnut
Strawberries
Capers Parsley
Blueberries
Kale
Citrus fruit
Medjool date
Turmeric
Buckwheat
Olive oil
Green tea
Soy.

Amazingly, coffee is also among this list of

Sirtfood diets. So, this is a great eye-opener, especially if you are a lover of caffeine. Japan and Italy are a few of the countries with very high Sirtfood intake. It is not a surprise that they are the healthiest country in the world.

Aside from these 20 Sirtfoods, which are featured mostly in the Sirtfood recipes in this book, we have an additional 20 recipes, which are fruits and vegetables. These additional recipes are very rich in sirtuin, thus making them activate sirtuins.

More so, these foods are prominent and very familiar recipes, and you may just have been making use of them if you love cooking food in your home.

More Sirtfood Rich Meals:

FRUITS

Plums
Apples
Citrus fruits
Red grapes
Blueberries
Cranberries
Raspberries
Blackberries
Goji berries
Black currants

VEGETABLES

Dill
Lovage
Artichokes
Chia seeds
Quinoa

Watercress
Spinach
Broccoli
Asparagus
Green beans
Shallots

THE DIET PHASES

There are two phases of the diet: one week, and the other is two weeks(14- day) plan, also known as the maintenance phase.

The first one-week phase involves taking a limited calorie of 1000 kcal for a maximum of three days. The diet consists of taking three Sirtfood green juice and one Sirtfood meal. The juice contents include Persil, citrus fruit, kale, rocket, green tea, and celery. For the Sirtfood meal, the diet comprises chicken and kale curry, turkey and garlic, creeping covered with buckwheat noodles of buckwheat, and caber and parsley. However, the other four days' diet is increased to 1500kcal and involves two Sirtfood green juices and two Sirtfood meals daily.

The diet also involves restricting food choices and the number of calories you should consume daily, especially at the starting phase. The diet also requires your water consumption.

The fourteen-day phase, also known as the maintenance phase, is marked primarily for weight loss because it occurs when weight loss occurs. According to Aaron, the second phase is a permanent and practical weight loss menu. But weight loss is not the only benefit the diet leverages; it also helps bring your table the best meals nature offers.

It includes three balanced Sirtfood meals and one green Sirtfood juice. Overall the Sirtfood diet bridges the gap between dysfunctional eating and diseases. It does not just function as a weight management meal but also enhances our health to ensure we live a longer and healthier life.

Starting The Process

In beginning the Sirtfood diet, you will require a lot of regular juices. To make things easier with making the juices get a juicer. There are also some very essential items you will need.

Also, go through the ingredients list to know the items you don't have to make buying them much easy. Also, ensure all the ingredients you need are not beyond reach. You can easily get powdered green tea like Matcha online or at the nearest health shop. The same goes for lovage, a green juice herb that can easily be acquired online. However, If it seems difficult, you can easily get the seed online and grow it in a pot.

Meal Advice

Eat meals on time. Your meals and juice intake should not exceed 7 p.m., which is the ideal mealtime. Also, take juice some two hours before or after meals to enhance absorption. Eat to your satisfaction, and don't get overfull. And lastly, enjoy every moment of your dieting journey, don't get all fuzzy in the process.

FOLLOWING THE SIRTFOOD DIET PLAN

Although the phases are divided into two, the maximum time for a Sirtfood diet is three weeks. So, it would help if you started using your diet now. However, the Sirtfood diet constitutes some sirtuin meals alongside some other components to give the 20 Sirtfood. However, buckwheat, matcha green tea powder, and lovage- which are the key ingredients for making these meals may be difficult or costly to find.

These twenty types of Sirtfood also have transforming abilities, which is why they are also known as a wonder food.

Health Benefit

The Sirt food diet has brought a whole new light on weight loss. Its focus has been how helping people access the best meal they can afford and are accessible to the meals they enjoy. This is all a Sirtfood Diet requires. It requires obtaining all the benefits of the meals. We are supposed to get in the right quantity and combination to bring the right body stature and healthiness we so greatly desire, transforming our entire life.

A Sirtfood diet does not require the traditional severe calorie cut back like other diet plans. Instead, it focuses on the meals you can include in your meals to give you a transformed lifestyle.

In a nutshell, the main functions of the Sirtfood diet are to:

Cut back body•fat by burning fat while your muscle is still intact. Prepare your body for a longer weight loss series and success.

DO SIRTUINS REALLY ENHANCES LEAN GENE

According to research, mice that have been induced with a high amount of SIRTI, the sirtuin causing gene has been observed to have a leaner build. Also, their body metabolism was more active than those without the gene. Those without the gene have more body metabolic disease and are consequently fatter.

Amazingly, when it comes to humans, the reverse is the case. Results have revealed that SIRTI is lower in the body of obese people, while people with lower genes are markedly leaner and more unlikely to gain weight.

Understanding this variance will bring to your knowledge why sirtuins are very good determinants to know whether we will stay lean or fat.

RECIPES

PHASE ONE RECIPE

MATCHA GREEN TEA

This particular Mocha requires sugar, so you can consider using unsweetened milk to tame the sweetness.

SERVE 2

Ingredients

2 teaspoons of sugar
1 cup of milk
2 cups of green tea or Matcha green tea
1 ½ teaspoon of unsweetened cocoa powder

Preparation

Pour the milk, cocoa, and sugar into a container and whisk until the cocoa and sugar are well dissolved. Then add a similar quantity of green tea into a mug or cup, and add the same quantity of the milk, cocoa and sugar mixture on it and serve.

It is great whether served hot or cold.

CELERY JUICE

SERVES 2

Ingredients

1 lemon, juiced
10 celery stalks with leaves, chopped
1 cup of clean water
2 tablespoon of fresh, peeled ginger

A pinch of salt

Preparations

Add all the ingredients into a blender and blend till it is well blended. Then strain out the juice using a mesh strainer. Pour into two glasses and serve instantly.

KALE AND ORANGE JUICE

SERVES 2

Ingredients

4 bunches of kale, fresh

6 oranges, peeled and cut into equal halves

Preparation

Using a juicer, extract the juice from the ingredients, pour it into the glasses, and serve.

APPLE AND CUCUMBER JUICE

SERVES 2

Ingredients

1 lemon, juiced

4 celery stalk, chopped

3 apples, cored and sliced

1 fresh ginger, peeled
3 medium-sized cucumber, sliced

Preparation

Using a juicer, extract all the juices from the ingredients according to the manufacturer's instructions.

Pour into the glasses and serve instantly.

MISO AND SESAME GLAZED TOFU WITH GINGER AND CHILI STIR-FRIED GREENS

SERVE 1

Ingredients

½ cup of red onion, chopped
1 teaspoon mirin
1 medium-sized celery stalk
1 small sized zucchini
⅕ ounce of tofu (blocked)

½ Thai chili

½ cup of kale, chopped

¼ tablespoon tamari

1 tablespoon of sesame seed

1 teaspoon fresh ginger, chopped

½ tablespoon olive oil

1 ½ garlic
½ cup of buckwheat

Preparations

Heat the oven to 400 degrees Fahrenheit, and cover a roasting pan with parchment paper.

Then, combine both miso and mirin and mix thoroughly. Cut the tofu into vertical halves and slice diagonally. After that, cover the tofu with the miso and mirin mixture and leave it to marinate while preparing the other ingredients.

Cut the celery, zucchini, red onion, ginger, garlic, and chill and leave it aside. Then cook kale for 5minutes, then use a steamer and set it aside.

Then put the tofu in a roasting pan, and sprinkle sesame seed on it. After that, roast it in the oven for 10 to 15 minutes until its color turns caramel.

Wash and boil the buckwheat with water in a pan alongside the turmeric, then drain it.

Using medium heat, fry the onion, garlic, chili, celery, and ginger in hot oil, fry for a minimum of 2 minutes on high heat, then reduce the heat to medium and fry for another three minutes or until the vegetable is evenly cooked and still crunchy.

Then pour the kale and tamari and cook it for another one minute. Serve with greens and buckwheat.

KALE AND RED ONION DAL
WITH BUCKWHEAT

SERVE 2

Ingredients

1 teaspoons of olive oil

½ cup red lentils

2 chopped Thai chili

3 garlic, chopped

4 ½ teaspoon coconut milk

4 teaspoon ground turmeric

2 teaspoon curry powder (you can use the medium or hot one if you choose)

½ cup kale

2 cups vegetable stock

2 teaspoon of mustard seed

2 teaspoon chopped ginger
½ cup of buckwheat

Preparation

Heat oil on medium heat in a saucepan and add the mustard seed. When the mustard seed starts popping, put the onion, chili, garlic, and ginger and cook for 10 minutes until it's all soft.

Add the curry and turmeric and cook for another 3 minutes, then add the vegetable stock and allow it to boil. Add the pencil and allow it to cook for another 25 to 30 minutes or until the lentils are evenly cooked, and you have a smooth dal.

Pour in the kale and coconut milk and cook for more 5 minutes. For the buckwheat, cook it with the remaining two spoons of turmeric and drain out the water.

Serve the buckwheat alongside the turmeric.

ASIAN SHRIMPS STIR-FRY WITH BUCKWHEAT NOODLES

SERVE 1

Ingredients

1 cup of chicken stock
1 Thai chili, chopped
3 ounce buckwheat noodles
3 garlic, chopped
1/ 2 cup green beans, chopped

¼ cup red onions, chopped

½ pounds large shrimp

1 tablespoon olive oil

I teaspoon chopped ginger

1 cup celery (leaves sliced and set aside)

1 tablespoon tamari

½ cup of kale

Preparation

Cook the shrimp in high heat in oil with tamari for 3 minutes. Set aside and cook the noodles in hot water for 7 minutes or as the package instructs. Drain and set aside.

After that, using a frying pan, fry the red onion, chili, garlic, celery (excepting the leaves), kale, ginger, and green beans on medium to high heat for 3 minutes. Then add the chicken stock and leave it to boil. Simmer it for about two minutes or until the vegetable is cooked but crunchy, not soft.

Then add the shrimp, celery leaves and noodles to the pan and boil for 3 minutes, then remove from the heat and serve.

PAN-FRIED SALMON FILLET WITH CARAMELIZED ENDIVE, ARUGULA&CELERY LEAF SALAD

SERVE 1

Ingredients

1 ½ tablespoon of capers

1 ⅘ ounce of arugula

½ peeled avocado, peeled, diced

⅛ red onion, sliced

1 tablespoon olive oil

1 tablespoon brown sugar

1 tablespoon celery leaves

½ cup cherry tomato, half

¼ cup parsley

1 garlic, chopped

1x 5-ounce skinless salmon fillet

¼ lemon, juiced

1 head of endive, halved

Preparation

Add the lemon juice, garlic, parsley, and oil into a blender and blend until it is thoroughly smooth. Divide the oil into two.

To make the salad, add the tomato, celery leaves, tomato, arugula, avocado, and red onion and mix them. After that, smear little oil all over the salmon and sear it in a heated pan for a minute or until it turns caramel on the outside.

Transfer the fish to an oven and allow it to bake until it is completely cooked. Clean the pan and reheat it on high heat, mix the brown sugar with the other half of the oil and rub it on the endive.

Place the cut part of the endive facing the hot pan and cook for 3 minutes, turning it at intervals until it becomes tender and evenly caramelized. Serve with the salad, salmon, and endive

BUTTERNUT SQUASH AND DATE TANGINE WITH BUCKWHEAT

SERVES 1

Ingredients

1x 14-ounce cans chopped tomatoes

2 Thai chili, chopped

I red onion, chopped

1 tablespoon of coriander, fresh and chopped

1 cups of butternuts, squashed, peeled and chopped

2 teaspoon ground cumin

1 ½ vegetable water

1 1/2 cup of buckwheat

½ cup of parsley, chopped

½ cup of Medjool date, chopped

I cinnamon stick
4 garlic

1 red onion, chopped

1 ½ tablespoon of olive oil

1 tablespoon of chopped ginger

1x14 ounce can of chickpeas

1 tablespoon of coriander

Preparation

Fry the onion, chili, ginger, and garlic in two t ½ tablespoon of oil for 3 minutes. Then place the cinnamon, a tablespoon of turmeric and cumin, and cook it for another 1 to 2 minutes.

Add the tomato, dates, chickpeas, and stock and let it simmer for 60 minutes. To get a thick and sticky consistency, add some water during this simmering period. It will also prevent the saucepan from running dry.

Then place the squash in a pan, and roast it(use a heated oven of 400oF) with remaining oil for 30 minutes until it's soft and has charred edges. Cook the tagine, and when it's almost ready, cook the buckwheat with the remaining turmeric according to the instructions given in the package.

Add the tagine and roasted squash with the parsley and coriander, serve it with the buckwheat.

BUCKWHEAT NOODLES IN A MISO BROTH WITH KALE, CELERY&TOFU

SERVES 1

Ingredients

I cup of celery, chopped
2 tablespoon miso paste
2 garlic, chopped
½ tablespoon sesame seeds
3-ounce buckwheat noodles
¼ cup of red onions

¼ cup of kale, chopped

1 teaspoon of tamari (optional)

1 tablespoon olive oil

1 ½ vegetable water

1 teaspoon of chopped ginger

4 ounce of tofu, chopped

Preparation

Pour the noodles into a pot of boiling water and cook on high heat for 6 to 8 minutes or according to the pack's instructions.

Add oil into a saucepan and heat it. Then add the onion, ginger, and garlic and allow it to fry on medium heat until it becomes soft, but not brown. Add the vegetable stock and miso and allow it to boil.

Also, add the celery and kale and let it simmer for 5 minutes. Don't allow the miso to boil as boiling it may spoil its taste and become grainy. If you desire, you can add some more stock if what you have is not enough.

Now it is time to add the sesame seed and noodles. Allow it to simmer a little then add the tofu. Serve in a bowl.

STRAWBERRY BUCKWHEAT TABBOULEH

SERVES 1

Ingredients

1 tablespoon olive oil
1 cup of avocado
1 tablespoon of caper

¼ red onion, chopped

½ cup of buckwheat

1-ounce arugula

⅛ cup of Medjool date, chopped

½ cupped of strawberries, hulled

2 teaspoon of ground turmeric

½ lemon, juiced

¼ cup tomato, chopped

Preparation

Boil the buckwheat with some turmeric according to the packet's instructions, then drain and allow it to cool. Mix the tomato, onions, parsley, caper, avocado, and date with the buckwheat. Then slice the strawberries and mix it in the salad along with the oil and lemon juice. Serve on top of the arugula.

BUCKWHEAT PASTA SALAD

SERVES 1

Ingredients

12 olives
A small handful of basil leaves
3 tablespoon of pine nuts
A big handful of arugula
2 ounce of buckwheat pasta
1 tablespoon olive oil
10 cherry tomato, halved

1 avocado, chopped

Preparation

With exception to the pine nut, add all the ingredients together on a plate. Then, sprinkle the pine nut on top.

WALDORF SALAD

SERVES 1

Ingredients

1 tablespoon virgin oil

1 ½ tablespoon red onions

1 cup of celery, including leaves and chopped

½ teaspoon mustard

1 tablespoon capers

½ apple, chopped

1 teaspoon vinegar

½ tablespoon parsley, chopped

2 ounces of endive leaves

¼ lemon, juiced

¼ cup of chopped red onions

2 ounces of arugula

Preparations

Mix the apple, onion, celery (and leaves), and walnuts with the capers and parsley. Then, whisk lemon juice, oil, mustard, and vinegar in a bowl to create the dressing. Make a base with celery and endive, and serve the apple mixture on it and add the lemon juice mixture to drizzle it.

SIRT SALAD

This super salad can be served in various ways according to the original Sirtfood diet. All you have to do is replace the salmon with other proteins you desire, whether tuna, chicken, or lentils. The choice is yours.

SERVES 1

Ingredients

⅛ cups of walnut, chopped
1 ½ ounce of endive leaves
2 ½ teaspoon of capers
½ cup of parsley, chopped

⅛ cups of red onions

4 ounces of smoked salmon, sliced

1 ½ ounce of arugula
1 ½ tablespoon of olive oil

1 Medjool date, pitted and chopped

¼ cup of avocado, peeled and sliced

¼ lemon, juiced

½ cup of celery, leave included and sliced

Preparations

Pour the salad leaves in a bowl or plate. Then, mix all the ingredients, and serve it on the leaves.

AROMATIC CHICKEN BREAST WITH KALE AND RED ONIONS AND A TOMATO AND CHILI SALSA

SERVE 1

Ingredients

½ cup of buckwheat
⅛ cup of red onion, chopped
1 tablespoon olive oil
⅘ chopped kale
½ pound of skinless, boneless chicken
2 teaspoon of turmeric
¼ lemon, juiced

I teaspoon of chopped ginger

To make the salsa, you will need

1 ½ tablespoon parsley, chopped
1 medium tomato, chopped
¼ lemon, juiced

1 tablespoon of chopped capers

1 Thai chili, chopped

Preparation

For the salsa, mix the tomato, chili, parsley, capers, and lemon juice. Then, marinate the chicken breast with a mixture of turmeric, lemon juice, and a little amount of oil and let it sit for 10 minutes.

Heat the frying pan until it's very hot, place the marinated sugar on it, and cook for a minute or until it gets a little golden on both sides. Transfer it to an oven and bake it for about 10 minutes until it's well cooked. Then, take it out of the oven and cover it using a foil. Let it stay for five minutes before serving.

While waiting, cook the kale for 5 minutes using a steamer. Add a little oil in a frying pan and fry the red onion and ginger until it becomes tender, but not brown. Then add the kale and fry together for another 1 minute.

Boil the buckwheat with the remaining turmeric and serve with the vegetable, salsa, and chicken.

TURKEY ESCALOPE WITH SAGE, CAPERS, AND PARSLEY AND SPICED CAULIFLOWER

Thin cuts are best, but if the turkey or steak you are using is too thick, you can pound using a meat tenderizer, rolling pin or a hammer to turn it into an escalope.

SERVES 1

Ingredients

1 tablespoon turmeric, ground

¼ cup red onion, chopped

1 cups cauliflower, chopped

1 Thai chili, chopped
2 ½ tablespoon virgin oil
2 garlic clove
2 teaspoon of capers

I tablespoon of dried sage

1 cup dried tomato, chopped

¼ cup of fresh parsley, chopped

½ pound turkey steaks

¼ lemon, juiced

Preparation

To prepare the cauliflower, pour it into a food processor and cut it using a knife until it looks like couscous.

Fry the red onion, chili pepper, garlic, and ginger in a teaspoon of oil until it becomes soft or tenderized, not brown. Then add the turmeric followed by the cauliflower and allow it to cook for 1 minute. Take out of the heat and add the tomato and about half of the parsley.

For the escalope, cover it with sage and some oil, and use the little oil left in the pan to heat it for about 6 minutes, while turning the sides. When it's thoroughly cooked, add the caper. Remaining parsley, lemon juice, and one tablespoon of water into the pan. This will become the sauce to serve along with the cauliflower.

SIRT OMELETE

SERVES 1

Ingredients

1 teaspoon olive oil
1 tablespoon of parsley, chopped
4 medium eggs
2 ounces of beacon

1 teaspoon ground turmeric

1½ ounce of red endive, sliced

Preparation

Cook the bacon on high heat, using a coated frying pan, till it becomes crispy. Do not cook the beacon with oil because it has enough fat to cook it. After that, clean the pan with a paper towel to remove any remaining fat.

Whisk the egg with the turmeric, endive, and parsley. Cut the cooked bacon and stir it along in the egg.

Add oil in the frying pan till it's hot, not smoking. Then pour the egg mixture into it. Using a spatula, move the uncooked egg around the pan until the omelet level becomes even. Lower the heat, and allow the omelet to become firm. Use the spatula to soften the edges and fold the omelet into half or roll up, depending on your choice, and serve.

HARRISA AND BAKED TOFU WITH CAULIFLOWER

SERVES 1

Ingredients

A pinch of grounded cumin
A pinch of ground coriander
1 Thai chili halved
I teaspoon chopped ginger
2 garlic
¼ red bell pepper
1 teaspoon olive oil

1 tablespoon turmeric

I teaspoon chopped ginger

1 ½ cup of cauliflower

¼ lemon, juiced

½ cup of parsley, chopped

7-ounce tofu, firm

1 cup dried tomato, chopped

Preparation

For making the harissa, cut the paper round to give you flat, round sizes. Take out the seeds and add to a roasting pan alongside one garlic. Mix with a little oil alongside the cumin and coriander and roast it in an oven (heated to 400oF or 200oC) for twenty minutes or until the pepper is soft, not very brown. Allow it to cool then blend it along with the lemon juice using a blender.

Cut the tofu vertically and slice it diagonally. Then pour it into a coated pan or line the one you have with parchment paper, then cover with harissa and roast it for twenty minutes with an oven.

Then place the cauliflower in a food processor until it is finely chopped looking like a couscous. If you don't have a food processor, you can use a knife to chop it neatly.

Mash the remaining garlic and fry it with ginger, red onion, and a teaspoon of oil until it becomes soft but not brown. After that, pour the turmeric and cauliflower and cook for another minute.

Turn off the heat, then add the dried tomato and parsley and stir. Serve with the baked tofu.

MUSHROOM AND TOFU SCRAMBLE

SERVES 1

Ingredients

1 Thai chili, sliced

1 teaspoon olive oil

3 ounce very firm tofu, chopped

3 tablespoon parsley, chopped

1 teaspoon curry powder

¼ cup kale, chopped

1 teaspoon of turmeric

½ cup of mushroom, sliced

¼ red onion, sliced

Preparation

Using a paper towel, wrap the tofu and place a heavy substance on top to help drain it.

Make a paste with the curry powder and turmeric with a little water. Then steam for 3 minutes.

Meanwhile, fry the onion, chili, and mushroom with oil in a frying pan over medium heat for 3 minutes until it becomes soft and brown. Add the tofu and other spice and cook till the tofu starts getting brown. Then, add the kale and cook for another one minute over medium heat.

Add the parsley, mix thoroughly, and serve.

TUSCAN BEANS STEW AND BUCKWHEAT NOODLES

SERVES 1

Ingredients

1 ½ teaspoon of tomato paste

½ carrot, peeled and chopped

½ cup of vegetable stock or water

1 teaspoon of herbes de Provence
¼ cup of red onions, chopped
½ cup celery, chopped
1 tablespoon, olive oil
½ canned mixed beans, drained
1x 14-ounce Italian tomato, chopped

2 garlic cloves
1 Thai chili, chopped

½ cup of buckwheat

¾ cups kale, chopped

I tablespoon chopped parsley

Preparation

Fry the onion, celery, carrot, chili garlic and herbs with oil on a medium heat using a saucepan. Fry until the onion becomes tender but not brown. Add the vegetable stock, tomato puree and tomato and boil. Then add the beans and let it boil for another thirty minutes.

Add the kale and cook until its tender, 10 minutes is enough, then add the parsley. After that, cook the buckwheat with the package instruction and drain. Serve the stew with the buckwheat.

CHAR-GRILLED BEEF WITH ONION RINGS, RED WINE JUS, KALE, GARLIC, AND HERB ROASTED POTATOES

SERVES 1

Ingredients

2-ounce kale, sliced
1 tablespoon of olive oil
1 teaspoon tomato paste
2 tablespoon parsley
3 tablespoon red wine
2 garlic, chopped
¼ cup of red onions, sliced into rings

Beef stock

½ cup of potatoes, peeled and diced

1 teaspoon cornflour, mixed with 1 tablespoon of water

1x5 ounce beef tenderloin
2-ounce kale, sliced

Preparation

Boil the potato for 4 to 5 minutes using a saucepan, and drain. Then place a small amount of oil in a pan and roast it for 45 minutes in an oven heated to 425oF or 220oC. Occasionally, turn the potatoes every 20 minutes to ensure its cooking evenly.

When thoroughly cooked, take out from the oven and sprinkle parsley on it and mix very well.

Add oil to a pan, fry the onion for 7 minutes until soft tender, and set aside to remain warm.

Using an ovenproof pan, heat it using high heat until it starts smoking. Then rum ½ teaspoon of oil on the meat and fry it on the pan over medium heat. When ready, remove the meat and set it aside. Pour wine into the pan to remove mead residue and simmer to reduce wine quantity, and until it becomes like syrup with a concentrated flavor.

Then, add the stock and tomato puree to the pan and allow it to boil. After that, include the cornflour paste for thickening, adding it bit by bit to maintain your desired consistency.

Serve with roasted potato, onion rings, kale, and red wine sauce.

SPICED SCRAMBLED EGGS

SERVES 1

Ingredients

3 medium egg

1 teaspoon olive oil

⅛ cup of milk

1 teaspoon ground turmeric

½ Thai chili, chopped

1 tablespoon of parsley, chopped

⅛ red onion, chopped

Preparation

Heat oil in a frying pan and fry the onion and chili until they become tender. Then combine the egg, turmeric, milk, and parsley and whisk it together. Pour the mixture into the hot pan and continue cooking on low to medium heat.

When frying, move the egg in the pan to prevent it from sticking or burning. Then serve.

ROASTED EGGPLANTS WEDGES WITH WALNUT AND PARSLEY PESTO AND TOMATO SALAD

SERVES 1

Ingredients

1 small eggplant, halved or quartered

1 teaspoon red wine vinegar

1 teaspoon balsamic vinegar

1 cup of parsley

1 tablespoon olive oil

3 tablespoon water

⅛ red onion, sliced

1 ½ ounce arugula

⅛ cup of parmesan cheese, grated

½ cup cherry tomato, sliced

¼ lemon, juiced

½ ounce of walnut

Preparation

Place the walnuts, olive oil, parsley, parmesan, and half of the lemon juice into a blender and blend till it becomes a smooth paste. Add a little water occasionally to get the right consistency, but it should be thick enough to stick to the eggplant.

Rub a little pesto on the eggplant and roast in an oven heated to 400oF, until it turns soft, moist and golden.

On the other side, cover the red wine with

vinegar and leave it aside. This will cause the onion to become soft and sweetened. Then drain.

Mix the tomato, arugula, and drained onion, then drizzle the balsamic vinegar over the salad and serve with the eggplant. Add the remaining pesto on top.

TOFU AND SHIITAKE MUSHROOM SOUP

SERVES 4

Ingredients

1x14 ounce firm tofu, chopped into cubes

½ ounce dried seaweed

½ cup of miso paste

1 Thai chili, chopped

1-quart vegetable stock

3 scallion, trimmed and diagonally sliced

7-ounce shiitake mushroom sliced

Preparation

Place the wakame in a bowl and soak with warm water for 10 minutes, then drain.

Boil the vegetable stock and add the mushroom and allow it simmer for 2 minutes. Then, dissolve the miso paste in a bowl with some amount of the warm stock, and ensure it is well dissolved. Then, add the tofu and miso to the rest of the stock, be careful not to allow the soup to boil as it will spoil the miso taste.

Finally, add the wakame, chili, and scallions and serve.

SMOKED SALMON PASTA WITH CHILI AND ARUGULA

SERVES 4

Ingredients

2 ounce of arugula

100ml of white wine

2 garlic, chopped

2 tablespoon olive oil

2 Thai chilies, chopped

9 ounces of smoked salmon, sliced

½ cup of parsley, chopped

11 ounce of buckwheat pasta

1 cup cherry tomato, halved

2 ½ tablespoon of capers

½ lemon, juiced

Preparation

Add 1 teaspoon of oil in a pan and heat over medium heat. Then add the onion, chili, and garlic and fry till tender, not brown. Add the tomato and allow it to cook for two minutes. Then include the red wine and bubble to lower it by half.

Cook the pasta with 1 teaspoon of oil for 8 minutes and drain.

Add the salmon, capers, parsley, lemon juice, and arugula to the tomatoes and mix. Then add the pasta, mix thoroughly, and serve immediately. You can drizzle the remaining oil on top of it.

SIRT CHILI CON CARNE

SERVES 4

Ingredients

1 tablespoon cocoa powder
3 teaspoon ground cumin
150 ml red wine
1 tablespoon tomato puree
1 tablespoon parsley, chopped
2 cups of beef stock
1 tablespoon turmeric, ground
1 red onion, chopped
2 Thai chili, chopped
1 cup of buckwheat
¾ cups of kidney beans
1 tablespoon coriander

2x14 ounce chopped tomato
1 pound lean ground beef
3 garlic, chopped
1 tablespoon olive oil
1 red bell pepper, remove seeds and chop

Preparation

Using a large frying pan, fry the onion, chili, and garlic for 3 minutes using medium heat. Then add the other spices and cook for two minutes more. Add the beef and cook for another 3 minutes over medium to high heat until it is evenly brown. Then add the red when, and bubble it to reduce the quantity to half.

Add the tomato, red pepper, tomato puree, kidney beans, cocoa, and the beef stock and let it simmer for 1 hour. Occasionally, you can add water to give it a thick and sticky consistency.

Then add the chopped herbs and stir.

Cook the buckwheat and serve alongside the chili

BUTTER BEANS AND MISO DIP WITH OATCAKES AND CELERY STICKS

SERVES 4

Ingredients

Oatcakes Celery sticks
1 tablespoon of brown miso paste
½ Thail chili, chopped
1 garlic, mashed
½ unwaxed lemon, juiced and grated
 3 tablespoon olive oil
4 medium scallion, trimmed and chopped

2x14 ounce cans of butter beans, rinsed and drained

Preparation

Combine the beans, miso paste, scallion, garlic, chili, lemon juice, and oil together and mash them till it becomes a coarse mixture. Then, serve as a dip alongside the oatcakes and celery stick.

KIDNEY BEANS MOLE WITH BAKED
POTATOES

SERVE 1

Ingredients

1 teaspoon ground sugar
1 teaspoon ground cumin
1 tablespoon olive oil
1 medium potato, baked
1 teaspoon turmeric, ground
1 Thai chili, chopped
⅛ red onion, chopped
1 garlic, chopped

1 teaspoon ground cumin

¾ cup chopped tomato, canned

A pinch of cinnamon

1 teaspoon of chopped ginger

A pinch of ground garlic
1 teaspoon of sesame
⅓ cup of red bell pepper, seed removed and chopped
2 ½ tablespoon parsley, chopped
1 tablespoon powdered cocoa
¾ canned kidney beans
150ml of vegetable stock
3 teaspoon of peanut butter

Preparations

Add the oil into the saucepan and fry the onion, chili, garlic, and ginger in a saucepan with medium heat for 10 minutes or till it becomes soft, not brown. Add the other spices and cook for 2 minutes more. Then, bake the potato in the oven heated to 400oF or 200oC for 60 minutes using a baking tray. Bake till it becomes soft in the middle, or crispy, whichever way you prefer.

Add the stock, tomato, sesame seed, kidney beans, sugar, red pepper, cocoa powder, and peanut pepper to a saucepan and simmer on low heat for 60 minutes. Then finally, sprinkle in the parsley.

Divide the potato to halve and add the mole on top to serve.

KALE CURRY AND CHICKEN WITH BOMBAY POTATOES

SERVE 1

Ingredients

2 cardamom sticks

2 ½ cups chicken stock

4 teaspoon turmeric

2 tablespoon mild curry powder

2 garlic

2 tablespoon olive oil

3 Thai chilies

1 stick of cinnamon

¼ cup of coconut milk

2 tablespoon coriander

4x6 boneless chicken, sliced to bits

1x14 ounce chopped tomato

1 tablespoon of chopped ginger

3 red onions, chopped

1 ½ cup of kale, chopped

1 ½ pound of potatoes

Preparation

Smear oil on the chicken and two tablespoons of turmeric, and allow it to marinate for 30 minutes. Then fry it for 5 minutes until it becomes evenly brown and thoroughly cooked through, remove from the pan, and set aside.

Add a teaspoon of oil on the frying pan and fry the onion, chili, ginger, and garlic over medium heat for 10 minutes. Fry till it is soft, add the curry and additional turmeric, then cook for an additional 2 minutes. Then add the tomatoes and let it cook for 2 minutes more. Add the stock, cardamom, stock, coconut milk, and cinnamon stick and simmer for 50 to 60 minutes.

Keep an eye on the pan regularly to avoid it from drying out or decide to add more stock.

Boil the chopped potatoes with the remaining turmeric for 5 minutes, then drain. Allow it to dry for 10 minutes, then place it on a roasting pan. Smear the remaining oil on it and roast for 30 minutes until it becomes brown and crispy. Rub it through the parsley when it's ready.

Add your kale to the simmering curry alongside the coriander, cook chicken, and cook for 5 minutes more until the chicken is cooked. Then, serve with the potatoes.

BAKED CHICKEN BREAST WITH WALNUT AND PARSLEY PESTO AND RED ONION SALAD

SERVES 1

Ingredients

1 tablespoon olive oil

¼ cup of parsley

1 teaspoon of balsamic vinegar

6 ounce of skinless bones

1 ounces arugula

1 tablespoon water

⅛ cup walnut

½ lemon, juiced

⅛ red onions, sliced

½ cup cherry tomatoes, cut into half

1 teaspoon red wine vinegar

1 teaspoon of parmesan cheese, grated

Preparations

For making the pest, add parmesan, olive oil, walnuts, parsley, half the lemon juice, and a little water in a blender and blend till you get a smooth paste. Add some more water until you get your desired consistency.

Marinate the chicken with 1 tablespoon of pesto and the remaining juice, and keep it in the fridge for thirty minutes.

Heat your oven to 400oF. Using an ovenproof frying pan, heat it on medium heat and fry the marinated chicken for 1 minute, turning both sides. Then place the pan in the oven, cook for 8 minutes, or until it is properly cooked.

Add the red wine vinegar into the onion, and marinate for about 10 minutes, and drain.

Add pesto to the cooked chicken as soon as you remove it from the oven and heat the pesto. Cover with a foil and allow it to rest for about 6 minutes before serving.

Mix the onion, tomato, and arugula with the balsamic vinegar and serve with the chicken. Spoon the remaining pesto on it.

SIRT BLUEBERRY PANCAKE

4 pancakes

Ingredients

1 cup of blueberry
6 eggs, whisked
1 teaspoon baking powder

½ cup oats

6 ripe bananas, chopped

¼ teaspoon of salt

2 tablespoon of olive oil

Preparations

Pour the oat in a blender and blend until it forms into fine oat flour. Then, add the baking powder, egg, flour, chopped banana, and salt, and blend till it forms a smooth paste.

Pour the mixture into a large bowl, and insert the blueberry. Allow the batter to sit for about 10 minutes.

Meanwhile, heat the oil in a frying pan on medium heat, then scoop two spoons of the pancake mixture into the pan, and spread to cover the pan bottom. Allow it to fry till it becomes golden, then flip to cook the other side. Serve hot.

MUSHROOM SCRAMBLED EGGS

SERVES 4

Ingredients

2 large-sized eggs

1 tablespoon olive oil

1 cup mushroom, finely sliced

1 teaspoon ground turmeric

1 tablespoon of chopped parsley

20g kale, chopped

1 teaspoon of mild curry powder

½ chili, sliced

Preparation

Add the turmeric, curry, and water in a bowl, and mix to get a light paste. Using a steamer, steam the kale for at most five minutes. Then set a pan with olive oil on medium heat, and add the mushroom and chili and fry for about 4 minutes or until it becomes tender.

Add the egg and the Tumeric and stir. Allow it to cook for two minutes, then add the chopped parsley, stir, and serve hot.

SIRT SMOKED SALMON OMELET

SERVE 1

Ingredients

1 large-sized egg
1 teaspoon olive oil
10g rocket, chopped
1 teaspoon chopped parsley
Smoked salmon, sliced
1 teaspoon of capers

Preparation

Whisk the egg in a large bowl. Then, add the capers, salmon, capers, and parsley into the egg bowl and stir together.

After that, add oil into a non-stick saucepan and heat on medium heat to get the oil hot, but not smoking. Pour the egg mixture into the pan and spread it evenly on the pan using a spatula. Cook until the omelet is well cooked.

Fold or roll the omelet with the spatula and serve.

PHASE TWO RECIPES

STRAWBERRY, CELERY & WATERMELON JUICE

This is another juice that requires the use of a juicer. Nonetheless, using a blender can also give you similar results.

SERVE 4

Ingredient

3 cups of chunky chopped watermelon

3 cups of strawberry
6 large celery stalk

Preparation

Combine the ingredients and juice it out. Mix and store in an airtight container to retain the flavor and keep in the refrigerator.

GREEN JUICE

This green juice is one of the trademarks of the original Sirtfood diet made by Aiden Goggins and Glen Matten. The diet has many sirtuin activators, but its preparation requires the use of a juicer, a device not common in many households.

SERVE 1

Ingredients

2 celery stalks

2 handful of kale

1 teaspoon fresh parsley

½ juiced lemon

½ small apple (green)

1 ½ handful of arugula

¼ inch of fresh ginger, chopped

1 teaspoon of Matcha green tea

Preparation

With exceptions to lemon and Matcha green tea, juice the rest ingredients one at a time using the juicer. For the lemon, either squeeze it by hand or use a juice, then add it to the other juice. After that, fill a glass halfway with the juice, then add your Matcha.

Whisk the combination thoroughly, then fill the glass with more juice and mix again.

INSTANT COCONUT ICED COFFEE

When taking a drink recipe that requires milk, you can use any type of milk. Also, soy stands as one of the best in the top 20 Sirtfood. So, ensure you have unsweetened, organic soy milk at hand every time. It is also a great way to include sirtuin activators into your beverages at all times.

SERVES 2

Ingredients

1 cups chilled milk

2 teaspoon instant coffee

1 teaspoon unsweetened cocoa

2 teaspoon sugar
I teaspoon vanilla

¼ cup walnut, grounded

Preparation

Pour all the ingredients into a blender and
blend till it becomes creamy. Serve chilled in a
glass.

SPICED APPLE GREEN TEA

Matcha green tea recipe is one of the most popular teas in the Sirtfood recipe. To make traditional Matcha, you have the special bamboo whisk. You can always order it online. But if it's not possible, you can use any tiny whisk you already have to take out the clumps from the tea.

SERVE 4

Ingredients

1 teaspoon of Matcha green tea
2 teaspoon honey
4 crushed cardamom pods
2 cinnamon sticks

4 cups fresh apple juice

1 medium chopped apple

1 teaspoon lemon zest

1 teaspoon of chopped or minced ginger root.

Preparation

Place the cardamom, ginger, honey, apple, cinnamon, and lemon zest in a large bowl and thoroughly mix. Pour the apple juice into a pot and warm on high heat until it starts boiling, then let it cool for five minutes.

Add the hot apple juice into the bowl containing the other ingredients and mix them.

Cover the bowl and allow the mixtures to steep for five minutes. And drain the mixture into a teapot using a fine-mesh sieve.

STRAWBERRY ICED GREEN TEA

For this tea, the strawberries used are chopped in chunks for a textured beverage. But if you intend to finish the entire drink in a day, you should consider crushing the strawberries into a puree.

SERVE 4

Ingredients

5 cups of water
3 cups of ice, crunched
1 teaspoon of lemon zest

5 tablespoon of Matcha green tea powder
1 ½ tablespoon of sugar (optional)
5 cups halved strawberries

Preparations

Boil water and leave it to cool for five minutes. Then place the Matcha tea in a large container, and add the hot water. Whisk them together until it is smooth.

Pour the lemon powder, sugar, strawberries, and broken ice into a large jug and mix thoroughly. Then add the tea into the jug and let it cool for about an hour in the refrigerator. Stir before serving.

MATCHA GREEN TEA CAPPUCCINO

For this recipe, in the absence of a frother or handheld blender, you can use a small whisk in generating some froth. The drink tastes wonderful with or without the froth, but adding some foam on the drinks adds some airy texture on the drink that tastes amazing when taken.

SERVE 2

Ingredients

5 tablespoon of Matcha powdered green tea
2 cups of water
2 cups of milk

Preparation

Boil water using a kettle and allow it to cool for five minutes. Then pour the milk in a pot and heat it on medium heat until it starts boiling a little.

Pour the Matcha tea in a jug and add the hot water to it. Mix them using a milk frother (electric), or a handheld blender until it becomes smooth and frothy.

Pour the Matcha tea into the two separate cups, equal amount. Then, add the warm milk into the blend until frothy.

Add the milk on top of the separate cup of Matcha and serve.

CREAMY GOLDEN HOT COCOA

This recipe may seem odd as it combines black pepper. But it helps to make absorbing the turmeric easier. You don't want to skip this recipe.

SERVE 3

Ingredients

5 teaspoon cocoa (sweetened)

½ teaspoon turmeric

3 cups of coconut milk

⅛ teaspoon black pepper

1 teaspoon of vanilla extract

½ teaspoon ground ginger

2-3 tablespoon of syrup or honey

⅛ teaspoon cinnamon (grounded) 1 pinch of salt

Preparation

Simmer a mixture of coconut milk, honey or syrup, and vanilla extract on a medium heat using a pot. Don't boil.

When simmering, add powdered cocoa, cinnamon, black pepper, turmeric, and salt, and whisk till it mixes well. Simmer for another 10 minutes, pour into a cup to serve.

GREEN SMOOTHIE

SERVE 2

Ingredients

1 medium handful kale
1 apple, chopped
1/2, lemon, juiced
1 medium handful parsley
1 cup blueberries

Preparations

Add all the ingredients into a blender and blend until it's smooth. Then serve.

BLACKCURRANT AND KALE SMOOTHIE

SERVE 2

Ingredients

1 banana, chopped

3 teaspoon honey

6 ice cubes, crushed

10 tender kale leave
1 sachet of powdered green tea

½ cup of blackcurrant

Preparation

Combine the green tea and honey in a large bowl and mix them thoroughly. Pour the mixture into a blender and add the other ingredients and blend. Serve cold.

MATCHA-BLUEBERRY SMOOTHIE

SERVINGS 4

Ingredients

1 cups of water

1 teaspoon Matcha green tea 1 cup rocket

1 cup kale, chopped

¼ lemon, juiced

1 cup of watercress

1 cup chopped parsley

1 cup blueberries

Preparation

With exception to the matcha powder, add all the other ingredients to the blender and blend until it becomes smooth.

Add the match and blend until it is thoroughly blended.

CHOCOLATE, BANANA & PROTEIN SMOOTHIE

When making smoothies, when you have both liquid and solid ingredients, add the liquid to the blender before adding the solids. It makes it easier to blend all ingredients thoroughly.

SERVE 2

Ingredients

1 ½ cup of milk
1 teaspoon flax meal (optional)
5 Medjool soaked date
1 banana, frozen

1½ tablespoon cocoa

½ cup of strawberries (frozen)

1 handful of kale (optional)
1 ½ cup of silken tofu

Preparations

Add all the ingredients into your blender and blend until the mixture becomes creamy and a little frothy.

CHERRY, BERRY & DATE SMOOTHIE

This smoothie recipe can be troubling because of the seeds in raspberry and blackberry. However, you can mash them to a puree and squeeze it through a strainer before blending them.

SERVE 2

Ingredients

1 cup of strawberries
4 Medjool dates-soak it.
1 cup of blackberries

1 cup of cherries

1 cups of Greek yogurts

1 cup of raspberries

2 cups of crushed ice

Preparation

Pour all the ingredients in a blender and blend till frothy. If you intend to remain it for later, then store it in a pitcher and blend again to combine it before drinking.

SPICED MOCHA JAVA

To make this recipe, you need instant coffee. But in the absence of instant coffee, you can use brewed coffee by exchanging 1 cup of milk with 1 cup of water you use for preparing your coffee. It results in a lower creamed mocha, but it's perfect if you are a coffee purist.

SERVE 2

Ingredients

2 ½ tablespoon cocoa powder

3 tablespoon sugar

1½ tablespoon instant coffee granules

2 cups of milk

⅛ teaspoon of salt

½ tablespoon brown sugar

¼ teaspoon cinnamon (grounded)

⅛ teaspoon cayenne pepper

⅛ teaspoon nutmeg (grounded)

Preparation

Add all the ingredients into a saucepan and cook with medium to low heat,a nd whisk for 2 to 3 minutes until it is warm, not hot. Serve using coffee cups.

SIRT MUESLI

Suppose you plan on making this recipe in a large quantity or need to make it before the next day. You can mix all the dry ingredients and store them in an airtight container. The next day, to use it, just add the strawberry and yogurt, and it is ready for consumption.

SERVE 1

Ingredients

½ cup strawberry, hulled and chopped

⅛ cup of buckwheat flakes

¼ cup of Medjool dates, pitted and chopped

¼ cups of buckwheat puffs

½ plain yogurt

⅛ cups walnut, chopped

1 tablespoon of cocoa nibs

Preparations

Mix all the ingredients and serve. If not consuming immediately, remove the yogurt and strawberries.

STRAWBERRY RED WINE SANGRIA

Most people are excited that the Sirtfood diet gives room for red wine, and this book will not be perfect without the sangria recipe. Increase the health benefits and flavor by introducing citrus and strawberries into it.

SERVE 7+

Ingredients

1 cups of water
1 cup of brandy
2-3 spoons of maple syrup
1 bottle of red wine

½ slice of orange

1 lime, sliced

1 cup of Grand Marinier

1 cup of strawberries

Preparation

Combine all ingredients with exception to sparkling water in a large pitcher or bowl. Then stir it thoroughly. Cover it and place it in the refrigerator for about four hours or more. This will give room for the flavors to saturate. Serve over ice, add the sparkling water, and stir it again.

OAT-BLACKCURRANT YOGURT SWIRL

SERVE 2

Ingredients

½ cup of blackcurrant

½ cup oat

½ cup of water

1 cup of natural yogurt

1 tablespoon sugar

Preparations

Combine the blackcurrant, sugar, water, and sugar in a saucepan under low heat and bring to a slow boil. Lower the heat and allow it to simmer for another five minutes, then remove the heat and allow it cool. You can refrigerate it until it is ready for use.

Mix the oats and the yogurt in a large bowl.

Serve by adding the blackcurrant mix in a bowl and adding the oat mixture on top. Using a cocktail stick, mix the blackcurrant and oat mixture and serve instantly.

YOGHURT WITH CHOPPED WALNUTS, MIXED BERRIES AND CHOCOLATE (DARK)

SERVES 1

Ingredients

⅓ cup of walnut, chopped
2 cups of mixed berries
1 tablespoon of dark chocolate, grated

½ cup of plain yogurts

Preparation

Add the berries into a bowl and add yogurts on top. Then, sprinkle the walnuts and chocolate on it.

Conclusion

A healthy leaving is essential, whether you are cutting weights or not. Not only are healthy diets essential, but it also helps increase longevity.

But with the introduction of Sirtfood, you can spend less time in the gym, or doing workouts and eat your favorite meals while slashing out excessive fats. What more can you ask for?

So, to provide you with energy, and other metabolic processes, the body uses the stored up fat, which leads to weight loss.

There are more benefits to using the Sirtfood diet as it helps you eat free and without guilt. Plus, the steps are easy and practical to follow.

Sirtfood diet is not just a way of eating; it is a

way of life!

Printed in Great Britain
by Amazon